PURE ALKALINE FRUIT WATER

40 PLUS FRUIT WATER RECIPES

BYRON LOVINGS

AuthorHouse™
1663 Liberty Drive
Bloomington, IN 47403
www.authorhouse.com
Phone: 1 (800) 839-8640

Published by AuthorHouse 04/27/2015

ISBN: 978-1-5049-0731-6 (sc)
ISBN: 978-1-5049-0732-3 (e)

Library of Congress Control Number: 2015906276

Print information available on the last page.

authorHOUSE®

Water is Life…

BOOK OPENING

The words 'fountain of youth' may be associated with being a fairytale to most, partially because the phrase have never been fully explained, but the word 'fountain' is referencing to the source of something, that source being the substance of life, the substance of life is water, yes, water maintain and sustain you(th). Not just any water, but pure water, water with a pH balance of 11.5 or higher. The fountain of youth is pure naturally alkalized spring water 13.5 pH or higher.

The body itself is eighty percent water, and when the internal body water or fluid becomes acidic, full of acid, the body regress against itself, and disease enter the body. It is a known fact that cancer can not exist in the body, unless the body is acutely acidic. Maintaining the body above the acidic level, and sustaining a higher pH level, constitute a disease free body, higher energy, good health, vitality, and longevity.

In food and water, the middle number for good and bad pH level is seven, everything beneath seven is acidic, and every thing above seven is alkalinity, which food and water beneath seven causes your body water to become acidic, or as we say toxified, which causes the body to age rapidly and deteriorate. Food and water above seven causes and increase life, and more abundantly. Alkalized food and water cause the body to feel youthful, pure energy, which is a mysterious feeling of energy.

If the body is acutely acidic, very toxic, and have been for years, the body will eventually succumb to its internal toxic state, it will develop toxic liver, toxic kidneys, cancer, diabetes, heart problems, lung problems, digestive problems, joint problems, lack of energy, bad vision, etc., etc., and most people will journey into the chemical field, seeking a solutions, which only toxicfy the body even more.

If you desire good health, youth, and great energy, you must detoxify your body, and detoxifying your body is a natural process. To detoxify means to remove poisons and toxins from your body, and to accomplish this, you must stop eating and drinking things that causes you to become toxic, you must eat and drink things that cleanse your body. You must also sweat as much as possible, because sweating remove tons of harmful toxins. Working out revigorate the body, but if you are unable to workout walking is good, walking at least 15 to 30 minutes a day, should causes you to break a good sweat. Before anyone engage in a workout, you should consult with a physician.

Stopping the intake of acidic foods and drinks is the first step to turning the body toward good health. Once we stop poisoning the body with acidic foods and drinks, we should began a diet of natural high alkalized foods and drinks. A consumption of natural foods only. At this point the journey have begun. Keep in mind, that as we decrease our acidic intake, we should have already been engaging in flushing and cleansing the body of all acids, poisons, and toxins.

A good body flush and cleansing is performed with naturally pure alkalized spring water, containing no chemicals, and haven't been purified through the process of chemicalization. For the greatest level of detoxing the body, you should infuse naturally pure alkalized spring water with added alkaline, and this is accomplished by adding fruit to the water, then allowing the water to sit for 2to 4 hours, before consumption.

After 2 to 4 hours the water is highly alkalized. The alkalized level of the water was increased by the alkaline within the fruit. It's official you have made naturally infused alkaline fruit water. Drink and enjoy with great pleasure. The water recommended for making 'alkalized fruit water' is a brand found at Walmart, Essentia Water, it is the only commercial water on the market that has been tested to have a pH level of 9.5, and it has no BPA in it's plastic container. Drink plenty of this water, and drink to good health.

Thanks for reading, and enjoy this book 'Pure Alkalized Fruit Water' and we hope that you achieve your goals of good health, for we all desire to attain good health if we have lost it.

THE HEALTH BENEFITS OF KEEPING HYDRATED

The human body is made-up of over 70% water. So it is understood that drinking plenty of water(fluids) to maintain and restore the human body natural water levels is vital for things like muscle functioning, joint functioning, and brain health, immune health, normal digestion, and yes even human mood. As you read further we have listed some major benefits of staying well-hydrated…

Water and water only will quench your thirst - minus the sugar found in sodas, fruit drinks, juices, and all other artificial sweetened and flavored beverages, and we have learned that sugar filled drinks only make us more thirsty. As we all know that sugar filled drinks do not flush toxins from human body, but add toxins to the human body. Water and fruits filled with water flush out the byproducts of the fat and other toxins. Drinking large amount of water also keeps your skin moist, your pores balanced, and skin soft and gentle —thus lessening your risk of developing skin problems and dry issues like dermatitis, skin winkling, and various infections, and other fluid deficiencies related illnesses.

Being hydrated is essential for keeping all muscles strong, lubricated, and energized with raw energy and strength. If you are wondering why, It is because H20 aids the facilitation of oxygen to your muscles so they are prepared when exerted. Being hydrated is also good for all of the functions of the human muscles. Reason being is because water assist the human body in regulating it's functions and brain function, it's also closely connected to balancing human moods and emotions.

When you perspire heavily or overheat; you loose body fluids, and these body fluids, which we know as sweat, assist in cooling the human body down, by coating the skin with what feels to us as water, this natural process of cooling the body, is within itself a method of maintaining a healthy temperature. But we must replace lost body fluids to assist our body in keeping itself cool. So we must be mindful of drinking enough Water, for it is essential for sweating and replenishing your water supply. The proper body fluid levels will increase and improve the blood flow and oxygen flow to your brain, which strengthening the cognitive function of the mind and increase memory.

The joints, spinal cord, eyes, and brain are surrounded and protected by pockets of fluid (water). When the body began to feel stiff it is usually related to lack of water. Sustaining proper fluid levels and staying hydrated is vital to their well being. Water assist the human body in eliminating bodily waste, making bowel movements and urination possible and easier, and excreting bodily waste that would poisoned the body and cause illensses.

Water creates and provide the ability for your body to easily digest foods—via the water is in your saliva and even within your digestive tract. We should see water as your secret weapon to fighting off illnesses, improving lymph fluid within your immune system, the substance which prevent headaches, joint stiffness, muscle weakness and fatigue, and also lightheadedness.

CONTENTS

LEMON LIME MINT ALKALINE FRUIT WATER

Ingredients:

1 gallon of natural alkaline spring water
1 tbsp of manuka honey
½ handful of peppermint or spearmint sprigs
2 lemons, sliced
2 limes, sliced
1 grape fruit, sliced
1 orange, sliced

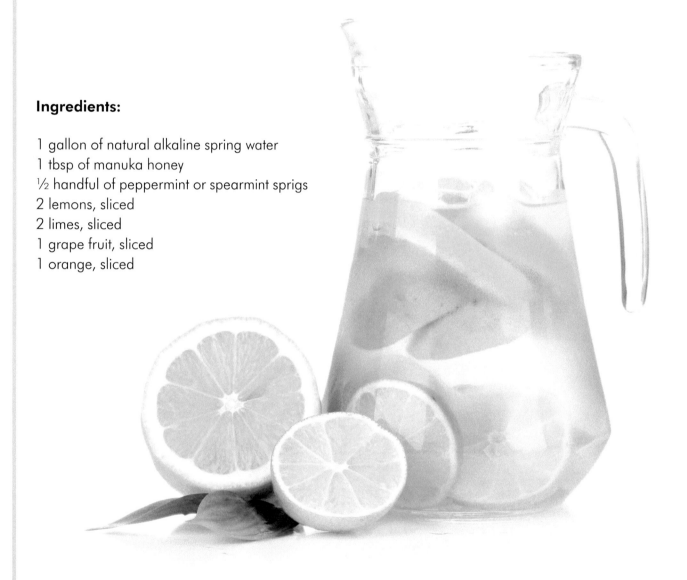

Directions: cut orange and grape fruit in half, squeeze them, pour juice into pitcher, add honey and water, stir, slice lemon and lime add into mix, add mint, serve immediate, but if you desire for the lemon and lime and other fruit to infuse into the water, allow the mix to sit at room temperature for 2 to 4 hour, then serve.

Great for body detox, hydration, balancing the pH, kidney cleanser, fat burner, and a great source of natural vitamin C.

A RECIPE FOR FAT FLUSH WATER (LITERALLY FLUSHES FAT)

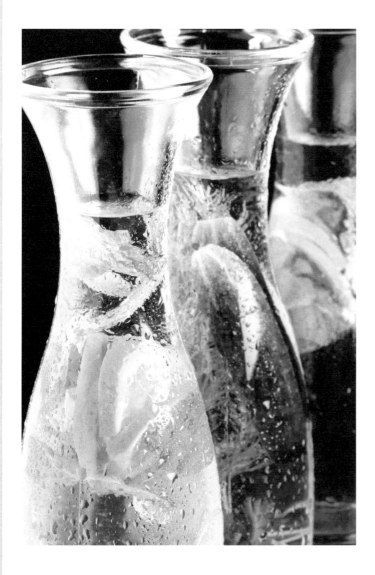

Ingredients:

1 gallon of natural alkalized spring water
1 tangerine, sectioned
1/2 grapefruit, sliced
1 cucumber, sliced
10 to 12 peppermint or spearmint sprigs
Ice, made from natural alkalized spring water
1 lemon, juiced and sliced
1 tsp. apple cider vinegar
1 tsp. aloe vera
1 tsp. honey is optional for sweetener and antibiotic

Place all ingredient in gallon sized water pitcher, allow the mix to sit at room temperature for 2 to 4 hours, stir, then serve over ice.

The tangerine increases your sensitivity to insulin, stabilizes blood sugar and because they are high in vitamin C, tangerine also boost the immune system, it assist to increase the fat burning process during exercise.

CITRUS REFRESHER AND LIME, CUCUMBER AND MINT

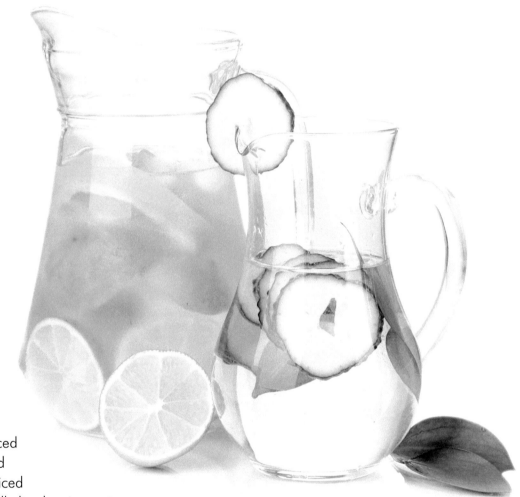

Ingredients

Citrus Refresher

1 lemon, thinly sliced
1 lime, thinly sliced
1 orange, thinly sliced
1.5 litres natural alkalized spring water

Lime, Cucumber and Mint

1 lime, thinly sliced
7.5cm piece cucumber, peeled, halved lengthways and finely sliced
6 to8 peppermint or spearmint sprigs
1.5 litres of natural alkalized spring water

Place all ingredient in water pitcher, allow the mix to sit at room temperature for 2 to 4 hours, stir, then serve over ice.

LEMON FRUIT WATER DETOXER

Ingredients:

2 lemons
6-8 peppermint or spearmint sprigs
1gallon of natural alkalized spring water

Directions: Place all ingredient in gallon sized water pitcher, allow the mix to sit at room temperature for 2 to 4 hours, stir, then serve, enjoy. After water have been alkalized, this drink would taste more refreshing after being chilled

Lemons is a great detoxer, lemons cleanses the kidneys, and rid the body of harmful toxins. Mint reduces pain, reduces digestive diseases, allergies, sore throat, and common colds. Both mint and lemons prevent diseases such as cancer and diabetes.

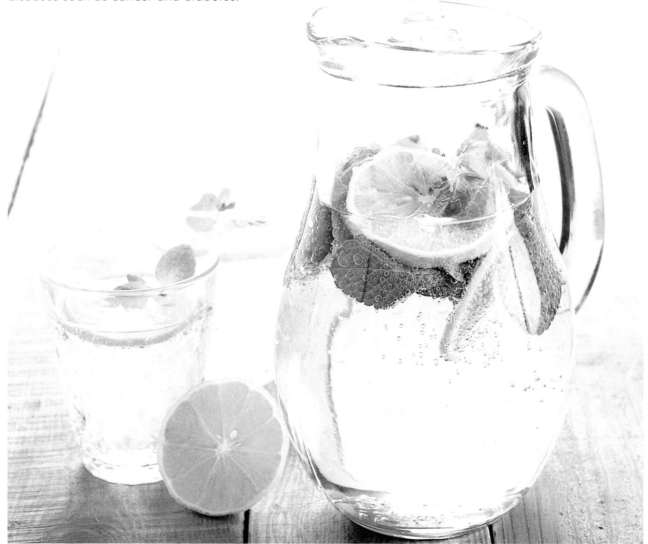

RASPBERRY PEACH KIWI ALKALIZED FRUIT WATER

Ingredients:

1 cup of raspberries
2 kiwi, sliced, peeled
4 peaches, sliced, unpeeled
1 gallon of natural alkalized spring water

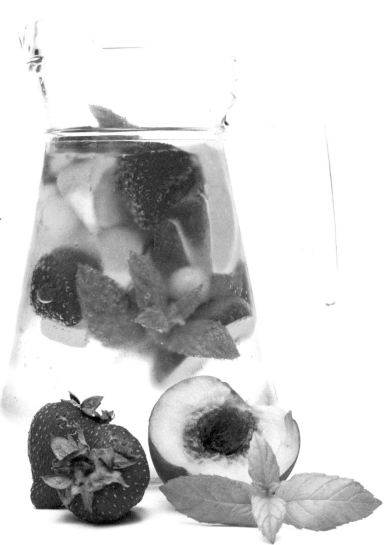

Place all ingredient in gallon sized water pitcher, allow the mix to sit at room temperature for 2 to 4 hours, stir, then serve, enjoy.

Health Benefits of raspberries;

Raspberries have significantly high levels of phenolic flavonoid phytochemicals such as anthocyanins, ellagic acid (tannin), quercetin, gallic acid, cyanidins, pelargonidins, catechins, kaempferol and salicylic acid… Scientific studies show that the antioxidant compounds in these berries play potential role against cancer, aging, inflammation, and neuro-degenerative diseases.

STRAWBERRY AND PINEAPPLE FRUIT WATER

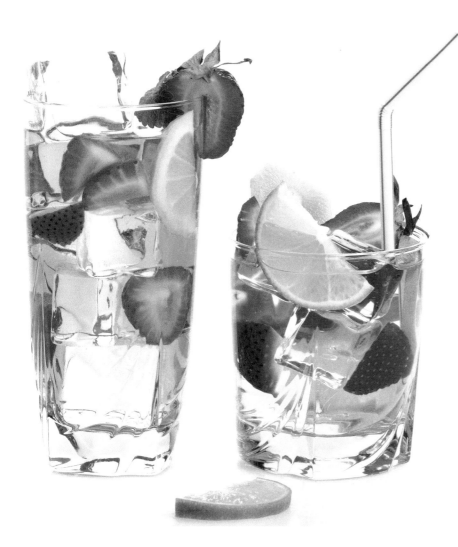

Ingredients:

2 cups of strawberries
2 pineapples
½ tsp cinnamon
2 tbsp of manuka honey
1 gallon of natural alkalized spring water

Place all ingredient in gallon sized water pitcher, allow the mix to sit at room temperature for 2 to 4 hours, stir, then serve over ice. Garnish with sliced lemons

The health benefits of strawberries;

Researchers have recently discovered that eating about 39 strawberries a day can significantly reduce diabetic complications such as kidney disease and neuropathy. The study showed that fisetin, a flavonoid contained in abundance in strawberries, promoted survival of neurons grown in culture and enhanced memory in healthy mice, along with prevention of both kidney and brain complications in diabetic mice.

ORANGE LEMON LIME AND BASIL ALKALIZED FRUIT WATER

Ingredients:

1 gallon of natural alkalized spring water
2 oranges, sliced
2 lemons, sliced
1 lime, sliced
8 to 14 basils

Direction: Place all ingredient in gallon sized water pitcher, allow the mix to sit at room temperature for 2 to 4 hours, stir, then serve and enjoy.

The health benefits of oranges;Oranges also contain thiamin, riboflavin, niacin, vitamin B-6, folate, pantothenic acid, phosphorus, magnesium, manganese, selenium and copper. Because of their high vitamin C content (over twice the daily need) oranges are associated with boosting the immune system.

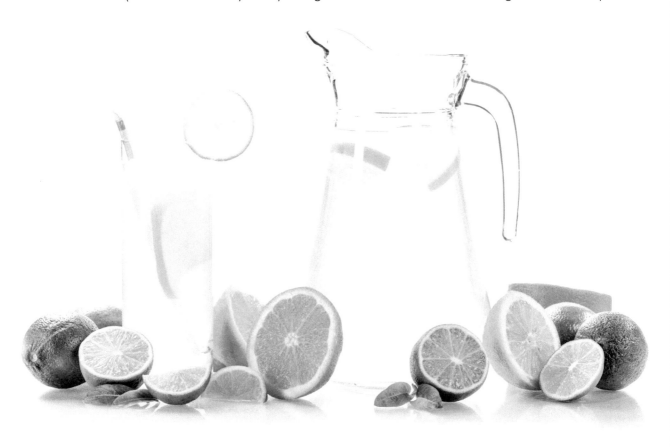

KIWI AND STRAWBERRY ALKALINE FRUIT WATER

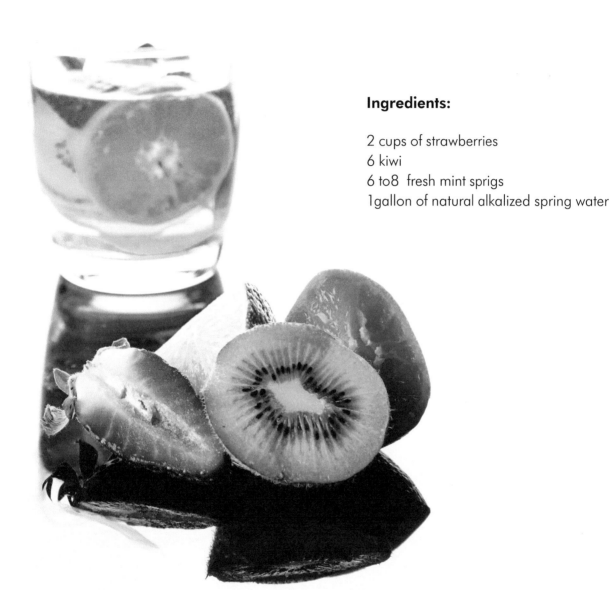

Ingredients:

2 cups of strawberries
6 kiwi
6 to8 fresh mint sprigs
1gallon of natural alkalized spring water

Directions: Slice kiwi fruit in to round shapes (width wise) Slice strawberries and take off the tops. Make slices of the strawberries. If you would like add a few mint sprigs. Fill your favorite pitcher with natural alkalized spring water and place the strawberries, kiwi's and mint. allow to the mix to sit for 4 hours to allow the flavors of the fruit to infuse the water. Fill glasses with ice and serve. For an added touch garnish the glasses with mint sprigs or sliced fruit.

FRUIT INFUSED COCONUT WATER

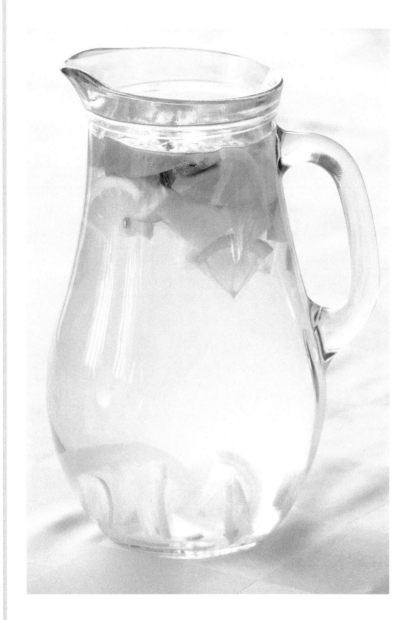

Ingredients

32 oz coconut water
1 orange- washed and thinly sliced
1 lime- washed and thinly sliced

Directions

Pour the coconut water into a pitcher and add the fruit slices, squeezing slightly to release some of the juices. Let the juice sit for at least least 2 hours but not more than 4 to 6 hours, the rinds of the fruit can make the Coconut water bitter if left in too long.

* You can add this mixture to a smoothie in place of the water or milk for a super hydrating drink!

HERBAL ALKALIZED FRUIT WATER

Ingredients:

Gallon of natural alkalized spring water
1 cucumber, sliced
1 lemon, sliced
8 sprigs of peppermint or spearmint
2 sprigs (each 2 in. long) fresh rosemary, slightly crushed

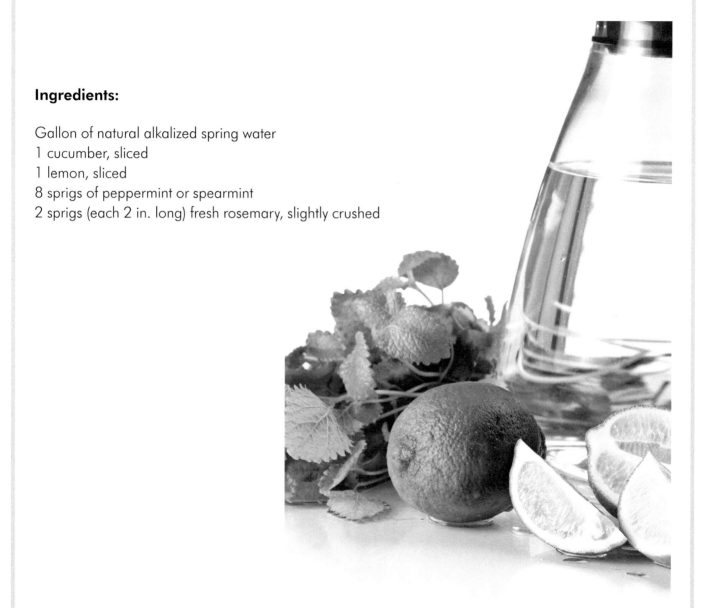

Directions: Place all ingredient in gallon sized water pitcher, allow the mix to sit at room temperature for 2 to 4 hours, stir, then serve, enjoy.

The health benefits of lime; The peels of citrus fruits contain an inhibit or of melanin production. The limonoid compounds in limes have been shown to prevent cancers of the colon, stomach and blood. Though the exact mechanism is unknown, scientists have observed that antioxidant limonoids also cause cancer cell death. Lime juice can help prevent formation of kidney stone. Fresh or from concentrate, lime juice contains more citric acid than orange or grapefruit juice. Citric acid is a natural inhibitor of kidney stones made of crystallized calcium.

CUCUMBER AND LEMON ALKALIZED WATER

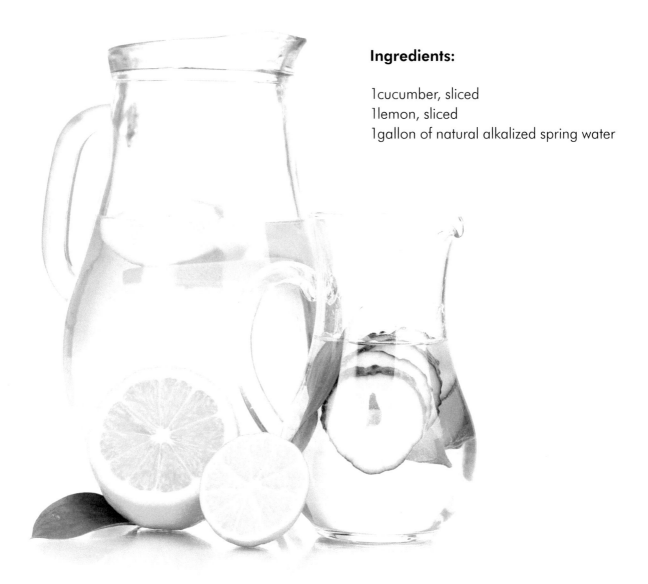

Ingredients:

1cucumber, sliced
1lemon, sliced
1gallon of natural alkalized spring water

Direction; Place all ingredient in gallon sized water pitcher, allow the mix to sit at room temperature for 2 to 4 hours, stir, then serve, enjoy.

One cup of cucumber provides 11% of vitamin K, 4% of vitamin C, magnesium, potassium and manganese and 2% of vitamin A, thiamin, riboflavin, B-6, folate, pantothenic acid, calcium, iron, phosphorus, zinc and copper needs for the day.

GRAPEFRUIT AND TANGERINE ALKALIZED FRUIT WATER

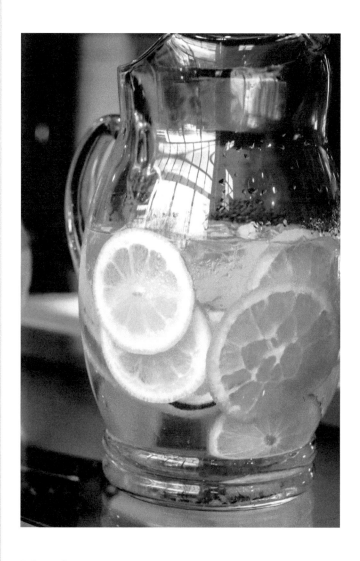

Ingredients:

1 gallon of natural alkalized spring water
1 grapefruit, sliced
1 tangerine, sectioned
½ cucumber, sliced
4 peppermint sprigs
Ice – as much as you like

Directions:

Wash grapefruit, tangerine cucumber and peppermint sprigs.

Slice cucumber, grapefruit and tangerine (or peel).

Combine all ingredients (fruits, vegetables, 8 oz water, and ice) into a large pitcher.

After Placing all ingredient in gallon sized water pitcher, allow the mix to sit at room temperature for 2 to 4 hours, stir, then serve, enjoy.

BLUEBERRY BLACKBERRY FRUIT WATER

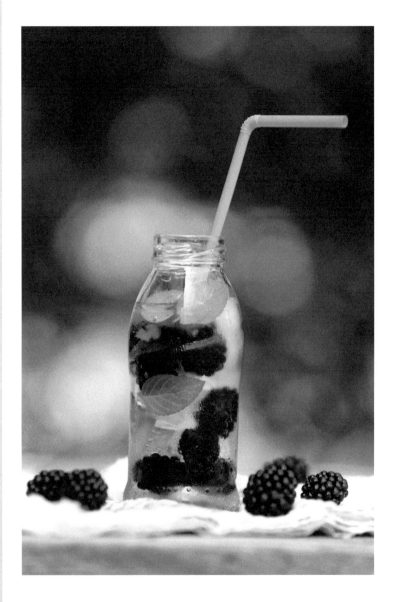

Ingredients:

1 gallon of natural alkalized spring water
1 cup of blackberries
1 cup of blueberries

Place all ingredient in gallon sized water pitcher, allow the mix to sit at room temperature for 2 to 4 hours, stir, then serve on ice, enjoy.

Health benefits of blackberry include better digestive health, strengthened immune defense, healthy functioning of heart, prevention of cancer and relief from endothelial dysfunction. Blackberry provides cognitive benefits and aids in enhancing memory, weight management, keeping the bones strong, healthy skin, improved vision and disease-free eyes, and normal blood clotting.

ROSEMARY AND THYMES
FRUIT WATER

Ingredients

1 gallon of natural alkalized spring water
1 cucumber
1 lemon
2 sprigs of rosemary
1 handful thyme
1 handful mint

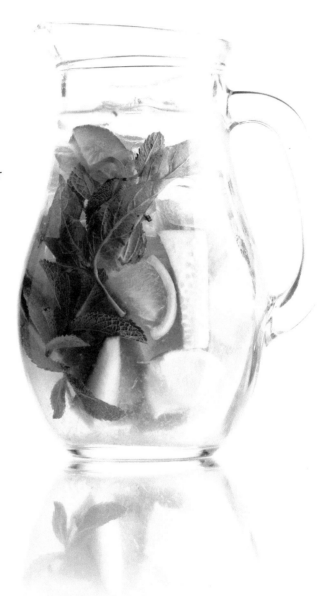

Directions: Place all ingredient in gallon sized water pitcher, allow the mix to sit at room temperature for 2 to 4 hours, stir, then serve and enjoy.

Rosemary contains carnosol which has been found in studies to be a potent anti-cancer compound. Researchers have had promising results in studies of its efficacy against breast cancer, prostate cancer, colon cancer, leukemia, and skin cancer. In one study, researchers gave powdered rosemary to rats for two weeks and found that it reduced the binding of the carcinogen given to the rats by 76% and significantly inhibited the formation of breast tumors.

LEMON LIME ALKALIZED FRUIT WATER

Ingredients:

1gallon of natural alkalized spring water
2 lemon, sliced
2 lime, sliced

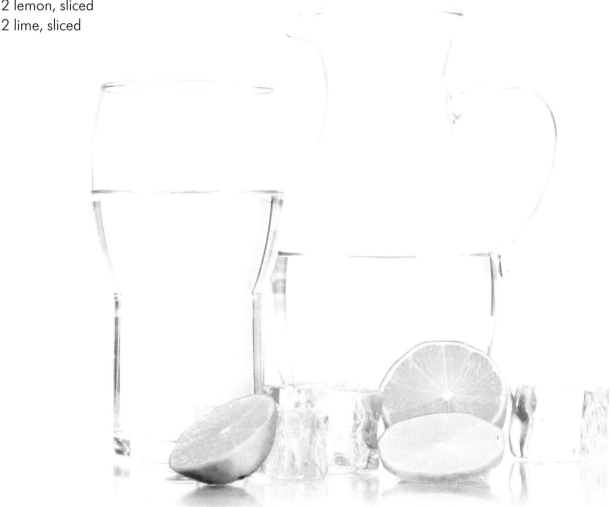

Slice lemons and limes, place all ingredient in gallon sized water pitcher, allow the mix to sit at room temperature for 2 to 4 hours, stir, then serve and enjoy.

The benefits of lemon and lime;

Limes and lemons contain outstanding phytochemicals that are high in anti-oxidant and anti-cancer properties. They are potent detoxifiers with anti-biotic effect that is protective against bacterial poisoning.

A SUMMER REFRESHER (AGUA FRESH)

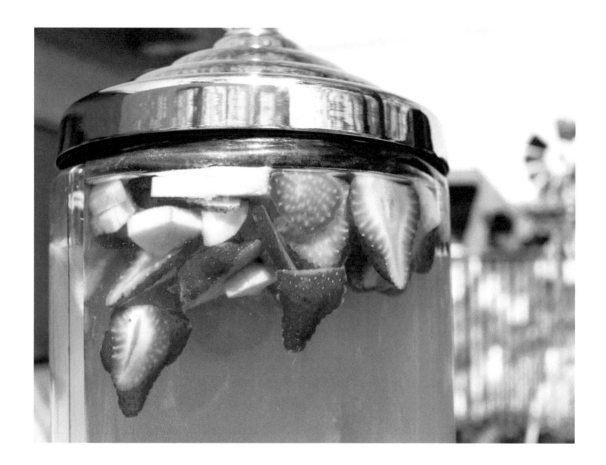

Ingredients

1 gallon of natural alkalized water
½ seedless cucumber, sliced
1 pint strawberries, sliced
1 small pink grapefruit, sliced

Place all ingredient in gallon sized water pitcher, allow the mix to sit at room temperature for 2 to 4 hours, stir, then serve and enjoy.

The health benefits of grape fruit;

The fruit contains very good levels of vitamin-A (provides about 1150 IU per 100g), and flavonoid antioxidants such as naringenin, and naringin. Additionally, it is a moderate source of lycopene, beta-carotene, xanthin and lutein. Studies suggest that these compounds have antioxidant properties and are essential for vision. The total antioxidant strength measured in terms of oxygen radical absorbance capacity (ORAC) of grapefruit is 1548 μmol TE/100 g.

CUCUMBER ALKALIZED WATER

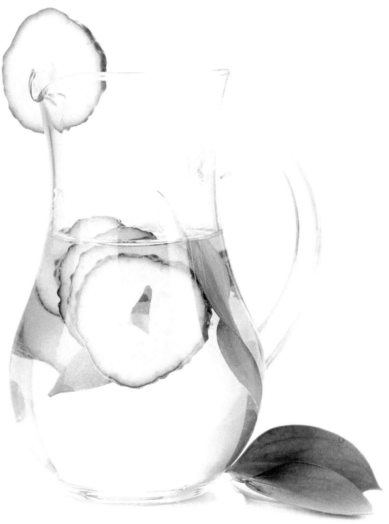

Ingredients:

1 gallon if natural alkalized spring water
2 cucumber
8 to12 basil leaves

Directions: Place all ingredient in gallon sized water pitcher, allow the mix to sit at room temperature for 2 to 4 hours, stir, then serve and enjoy.

Basil herb contains many polyphenolic flavonoids like orientin and vicenin. These compounds were tested in-vitro laboratory for their possible anti-oxidant protection against radiation-induced lipid per-oxidation in mouse liver. Basil leaves compose of several health benefiting essential oils such as eugenol, citronellol, linalool, citral, limonene and terpineol. These compounds are known to have anti-inflammatory and anti-bacterial properties.

MINT LEMON RASPBERRY ALKALIZED FRUIT WATER

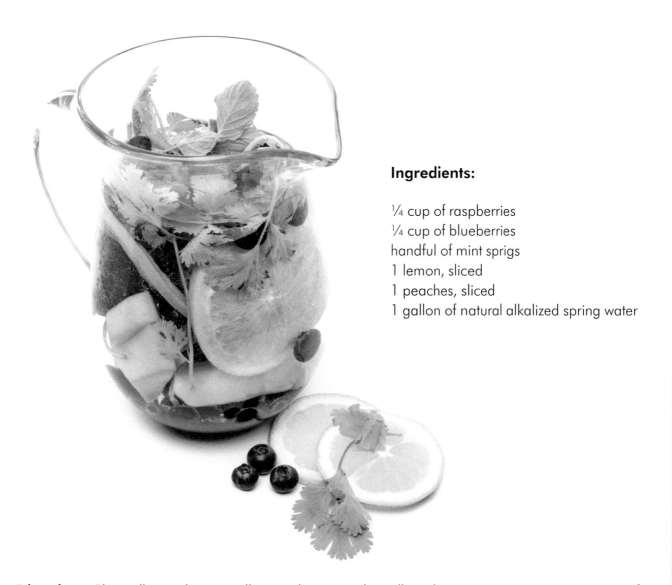

Ingredients:

¼ cup of raspberries
¼ cup of blueberries
handful of mint sprigs
1 lemon, sliced
1 peaches, sliced
1 gallon of natural alkalized spring water

Directions: Place all ingredient in gallon sized water pitcher, allow the mix to sit at room temperature for 2 to 4 hours, stir, then serve and enjoy.

Fresh peaches are a moderate source of antioxidant, vitamin-C. Vitamin-C has anti-oxidant effects and is required for connective tissue synthesis inside the human body. Consumption of foods rich in vitamin C helps develop resistance against infectious agents, and help scavenges harmful free radicals. Fresh fruits are also a moderate source of vitamin-A and ß-carotene. ß-carotene is a pro-vitamin, which converts into vitamin A inside the body. Vitamin A is essential for night vision. It is also essential for maintaining healthy mucus membranes and skin. Consumption of natural fruits rich in vitamin A is known to offer protection from lung and oral cavity cancers.

MINT LIME BLUEBERRY FRUIT WATER AND LEMON STRAWBERRY BASIL FRUIT WATER

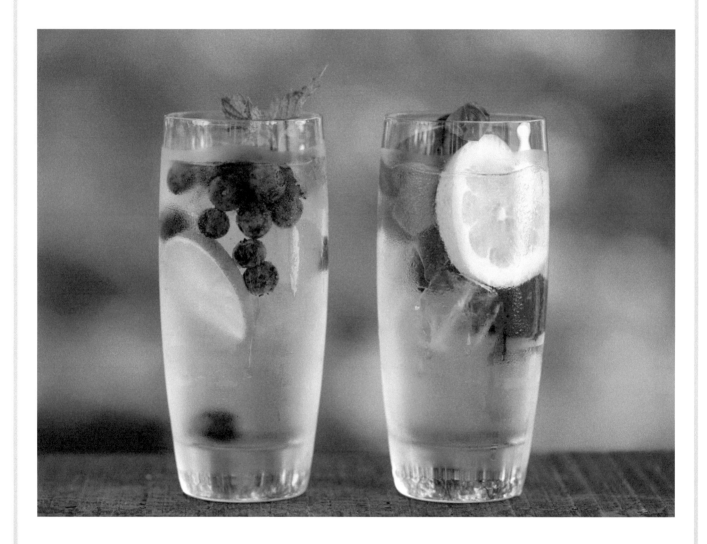

Mint Lime Blueberry Fruit Water

Ingredients:

1 gallon of natural alkalized spring water
cup of blue berries
2 lime, sliced
handful of mint leaves

Lemon Strawberry Basil Fruit Water

1 gallon of natural alkalized spring water
cup of strawberries
2 lemons, sliced
handful of mint leaves

STRAWBERRY KIWI LIME ALKALIZED FRUIT WATER

Ingredients:

½ litre of natural alkalized spring water
½ litre of natural ginger ale (no high fructose corn syrup)
2 kiwis, sliced
½ cup of raspberries
2 limes, sliced
4 tbsp of manuka honey

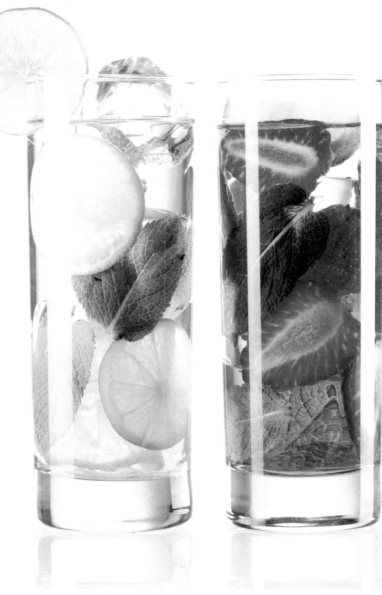

Directions: Place all ingredient in gallon sized water pitcher, allow the mix to sit at room temperature for 2 to 4 hours, stir, then serve and enjoy.

Kiwifruit is a nutrient-dense fruit that only provides 90 calories per 148-gram serving, most of which come from the 20 grams of carbohydrates present in the fruit. A serving of kiwifruit also provides 4 grams, or 16 percent of the daily requirements, of dietary fiber, which helps to lower the risk of heart disease by decreasing blood cholesterol levels. While kiwifruit contains substantial amounts of vitamin C and folate, some of the other nutrients present in kiwifruit include potassium, magnesium, vitamin E and zinc.

MINT AND LIME ALKALIZED FRUIT WATER

Ingredients:

1 gallon of natural alkalized spring water
handful of peppermint or spearmint
2 limes, sliced

Directions: Place all ingredient in gallon sized water pitcher, allow the mix to sit at room temperature for 2 to 4 hours, stir, then serve and enjoy.

Two thirds of our body is made up of H20 but how does that actually break down?

*The blood that flows through your body and delivers nutrients is 82% water
*The muscles that hold your bones and move your body are 75% water
*Lungs that pump oxygen crucial to your survival are 90% water
*Bones that protect your organs are 25% water
*Your brain is a whopping 76% water

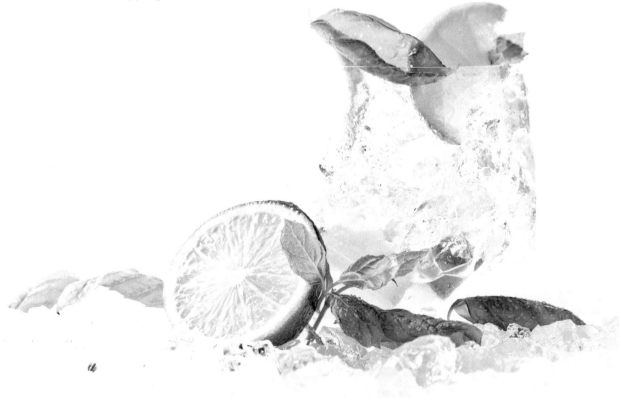

BAKING SODA - BASIL - GRAPEFRUIT ALKALIZED TONIC

Ingredient:

1 gallon of natural alkalized spring water
handful basil
½ ginger
2 grapefruit, pealed, sliced
2 tbsp of baking soda

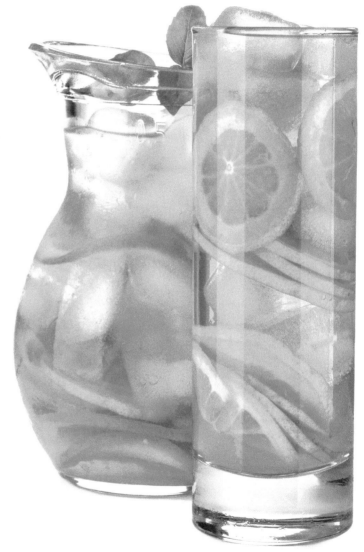

Direction: Place all ingredient in gallon sized water pitcher, allow the mix to sit at room temperature for 2 to 4 hours, stir, then serve and enjoy.

The benefits of ginger; Fights Common Respiratory Problems. If you're suffering from common respiratory diseases such as a cough, ginger aids in expanding your lungs and loosening up phlegm because it is a natural expectorant that breaks down and removes mucus.. That way you can quickly recover from difficulty in breathing.

POMEGRANATE BLOOD ORANGE PUNCH AND HERBAL WINE

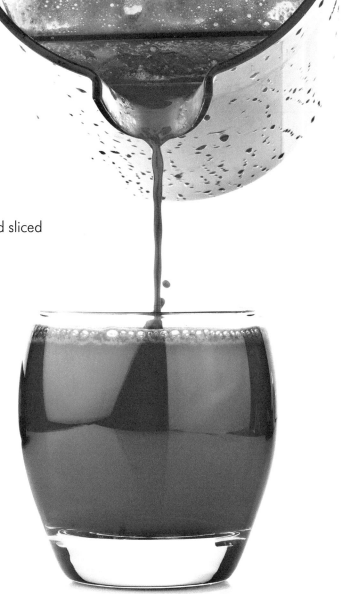

Ingredients:

1 orange
1 lemon
1 lime
1 medium all purpose apples, pared, cored and sliced
1 cup pitted cherries
1 cup fresh pineapple chunks
1 (750 ml) bottle herbal wine

Directions: Slice the orange, lemon, and lime into thin rounds and place them in a pitcher with the apples, cherries, and pineapple. Pour in the herbal wine and refrigerate for 2 hours of more. Chill the bottle of red wine, add ice to the pitcher, pour the wine into the pitcher. Gently crush the fruits with a spoon, then stir in the red herbal wine, add seven-up, and orange juice, for sweetener, and serve.

BLACKBERRY LEMON GINGER WATER

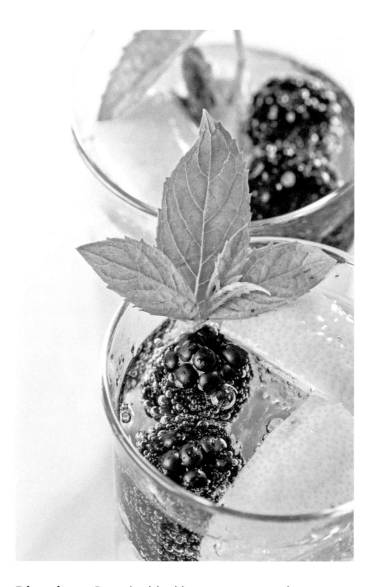

Ingredients:

½ pint blackberries, washed
1 knob of ginger
1 small lemon
4 cups of natural alkalized spring water
Ice, made from natural alkalized spring water

Directions: Pour the blackberries into a pitcher.

Wash the knob of ginger, then slice into thin slices, leaving the peel on.

Slice the lemon into thin slices. Put the ginger and lemon into the pitcher of blackberries. Fill with water.

Using the back of a wooden spoon gently smash some of the blackberries while stirring the water.

Let sit a room temperature for 2 to 4 hours.

Fill with ice, stir and enjoy.

THYME LEMON AND BAKING SODA INFUSED WATER

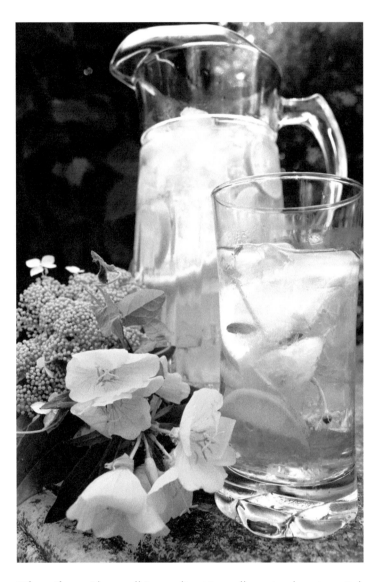

Ingredients:

pitcher of natural alkalized spring water
handful of thymes
2 lemons, sliced
2 tbsp of baking soda

Direction: Place all ingredient in gallon sized water pitcher, allow the mix to sit at room temperature for 2 to 4 hours, stir, then serve and enjoy.

Health Benefit of Baking Soda: Kidney Disease Bicarbonate is an alkaline substance naturally produced in the body that buffers acids and helps keep pH in check. In people who have chronic kidney disease, which is most often caused by diabetes or hypertension, poorly functioning kidneys have a hard time removing acid from the body. This often results in a condition known as metabolic acidosis.

BLUEBERRY AND STRAWBERRY FRUIT WATER

Ingredients:

1gallon of natural alkalized spring water
2 cups of blueberries
2 cups of strawberry

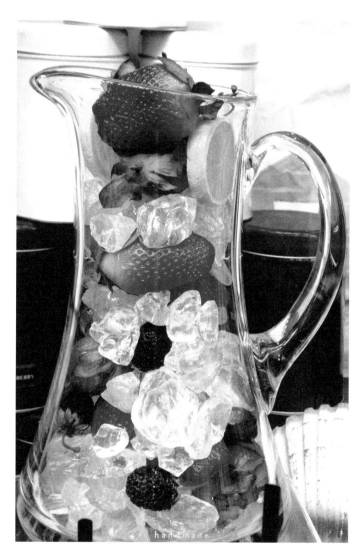

Place all ingredient in gallon sized water pitcher, allow the mix to sit at room temperature for 2 to 4 hours, stir, then serve on ice, add honey for sweetener, and enjoy.

alkaline water -

Definitions:

1. a water that contains appreciable amounts of the bicarbonates of calcium, lithium, potassium, or sodium.

CUCUMBER MINT ALKALIZED WATER

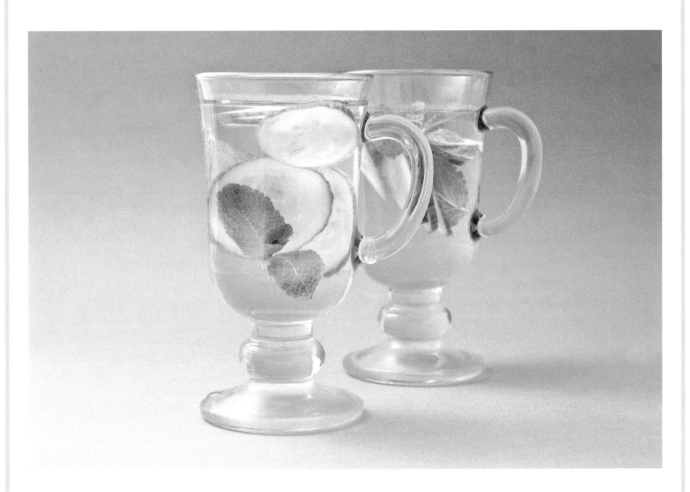

Ingredients:

1 cucumber, sliced
handful of fresh mint
pitcher of natural alkaline spring water

Place all ingredient in gallon sized water pitcher, allow the mix to sit at room temperature for 2 to 4 hours, stir, then serve and enjoy.

DID YOU KNOW..?

Keeping the body hydrated helps the heart more easily pump blood through the blood vessels to the muscles. And which helps the muscles work more efficiently.

WATERMELON COCONUT FRUIT WATER

Ingredients:

1 (3 pound) seedless watermelon, cubed
(about 5 cups)
4 cups (1 quart) coconut water
2 tablespoons freshly squeezed lime juice
(from 1 medium lime)

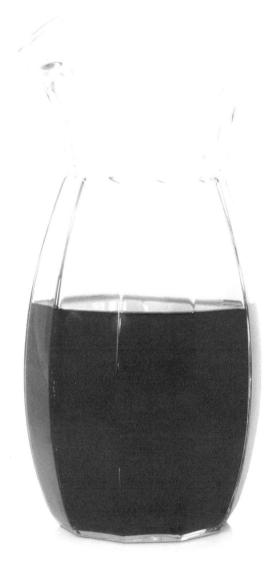

Directions:

Puree the watermelon in a blender. Place a fine-mesh sieve over a pitcher and carefully pour the pureed watermelon through the sieve. Discard pulp.

Stir in coconut water and lime juice.

Chill, covered, until cold - at least an hour. Serve over ice.

Watermelon, after being the brunt of so many jokes, have the highest pH level of all melons, and above all fruit, watermelon pH level is 12.5, and this level could heal the body of any ailment.

LEMON AND CILANTRO ALKALIZED FRUIT WATER

Ingredients:

gallon of natural alkalized spring water
1 cucumbers,
2 lemons,
½ cup of grapes
handful of cilantro, parsley
cup of frozen cranberries

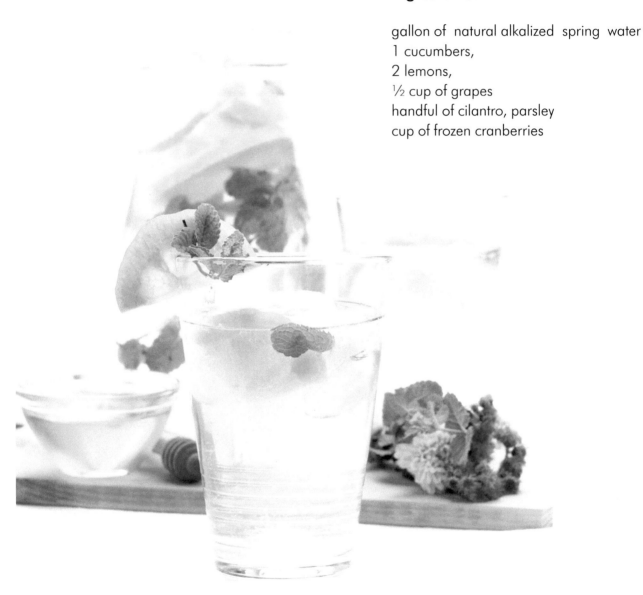

Direction: Place all ingredient in gallon sized water pitcher, allow the mix to sit at room temperature for 2 to 4 hours, stir, then serve and enjoy.

Great kidney flush! Great detox!

STRAWBERRY AND LIME ALKALIZED FRUIT WATER

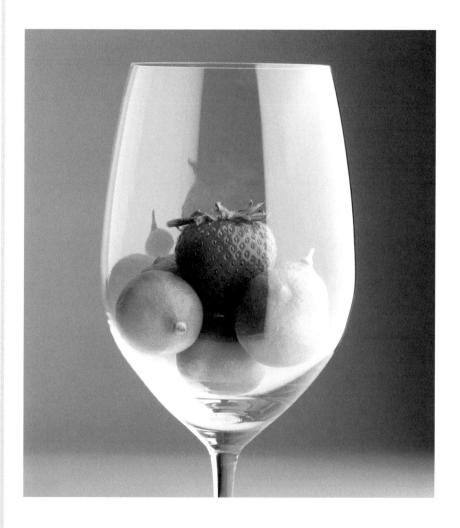

Ingredients:

1 gallon of natural alkaline
spring water
handful of mints
1 cucumber
cup of strawberries

Directions: Mix all ingredients in a jar, and let sit at room temperature for 2 to 4 hours, then serve, enjoy.

Healthy Tips:

To flush the liver, avoid animal products and eat mainly high-fibre fruits, vegetables, seeds, nuts, and legumes (see "Raw foods to support liver cleansing" below). Drink 6 to 12 cups (1.5 to 3 L) of filtered or healthy spring water daily because it helps flush out toxins. Avoid saturated fats, refined sugar, and alcohol. Enjoy vegetable juices such as beets, celery, and carrots, but do not focus the diet solely on these juices, as not everyone will find a juice-based cleanse to be convenient. If possible, make use of the far infrared sauna every two or three days to safely remove stored toxins from the body.

FLAVORED GINGER ALE WITH BLUEBERRIES, LEMON, LIME AND GINGER

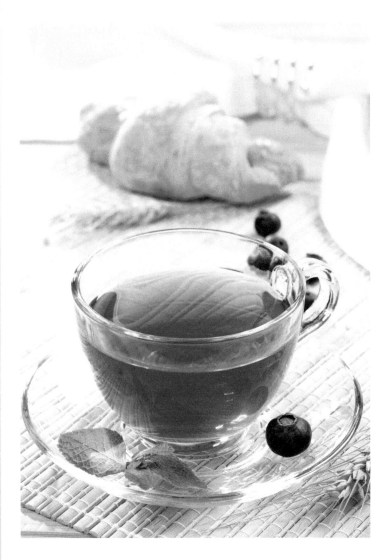

Ingredients

2 2 liter bottle naturally sweetened ginger ale, chilled
1 cup blueberries
1 lemon, thinly sliced
1 lime, thinly sliced
2 tablespoons crystallized ginger

Directions: Divide one bottle of the ginger ale between two half-gallon jars or pitchers. Add 1/2 cup of the berries, half the lemon slices, half the lime slices and 1 tablespoon of the ginger to each jar. Cover and refrigerate for 2 to 4 hours. (If chilling more than 2 hours, add the lemon and lime slices only 1 to 2 hours before serving. Citrus adds a slightly bitter flavor after 2 hours.)

Just before serving, fill jars with ice. To serve, fill each glass half full with the blueberry mixture and ice; fill glass with chilled ginger ale for fizz. Makes 12 servings.

RASPBERRY STRAWBERRY ALKALIZED FRUIT WATER

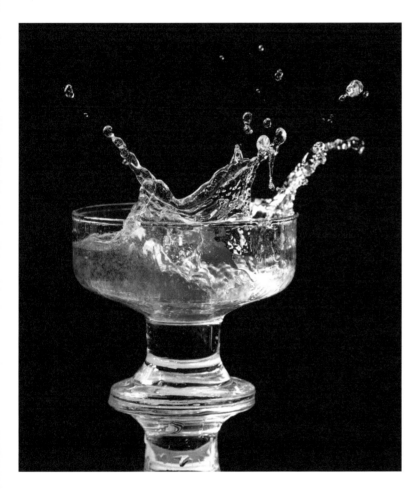

Ingredients:

jar of natural alkalized spring water
4 icecubes
about 10 raspberries
5 sliced strawberries – Adds a
wonderful flavor to the water

Instructions

In a glass – combine water and ice (about ¾th of the glass)

Add diced strawberries (about 3 small berries) and raspberries

Stir and left sit for 5 minutes – then enjoy! (The have anti-aging properties of strawberries -- perfect for naturally reversing the aging process)

Another combination rich in antioxidants – this one is simple, looks quenching, tastes amazing, and best of all can be reused! When finished with this infused water for the day strain the berries and place them into refrigerator to later add to a smoothie – this fiber content which is important for digestion.

HONEY GINGER AND LEMON ALKALIZED WATER

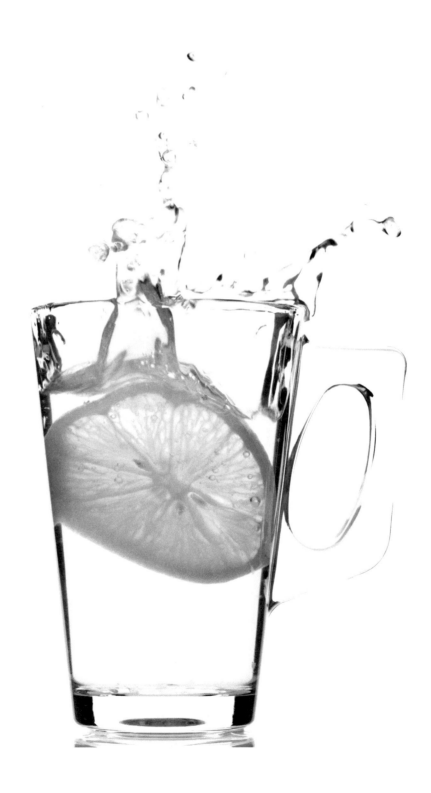

Ingredients:

For the honey ginger syrup:

1 cup (250ml) honey (I use wildflower honey)
1 cup (250ml) water (filtered or spring)
4oz (115g) fresh ginger root, peeled and finely grated (I use a microplane zester)

For the lemonade:

1 cup (250ml) fresh squeezed lemon juice, strained (about 5 large lemons)
3 cups (750ml) cold filtered or spring water (flat or sparkling)
1/2 cup (125ml) vodka (optional)
Ice for serving
Sliced lemons and mint sprigs for garnish (optional)

Directions:

To make the honey ginger syrup:

Place the honey and water in a medium saucepan, bring to a boil and simmer until honey is completely dissolved.

Turn off heat and add the freshly grated ginger and any juices. Cover and let steep for 30 minutes.

Strain syrup thorough a fine mesh sieve into a bowl, pressing hard on the ginger pulp and then discarding the solids.

Pour into a bottle or jar, let cool completely and then chill until cold, about 1 hour. The syrup will keep in your refrigerator for up to two weeks.

To make the lemonade:

Add the freshly squeezed lemon juice and the honey ginger syrup to a large pitcher.

Add 3 cups of cold water (more or less depending on how strong you like your lemonade). If you are using sparkling water don't add it until you are ready to serve so that it doesn't lose its fizz. Add the vodka now as well if using. Refrigerate until ready to serve.

Pour lemonade over ice filled glasses, top with a slice of lemon, and garnish with a sprig of mint.

WATERMELON LEMON RASPBERRY ALKALINE FRUIT WATER

Ingredients

2 lb/ 900g seedless watermelon, cubed (from about a small melon)
1 cup/140g fresh or frozen raspberries
1 cup/ 240ml freshly squeezed lemon juice (from about 8 lemons)
1 cup/240ml coconut water or filtered water (if using plain water you may want to add a little extra liquid sweetener like honey to taste if you like your lemonade on the sweeter side)
A pinch of sea salt or Himalayan salt (optional)
Crushed ice for serving
Slices of watermelon, raspberries and lemon wedges for garnish (optional)

Instructions

In a high speed blender or food processor, purée the watermelon, raspberries and lemon juice in until smooth. (You may need to do this in batches depending on the size of your blender or processor.)

Press through a fine mesh filter to strain and transfer to a large pitcher. Add the coconut water (or plain water if using) and stir to combine.

Refrigerate for at least 2 hours to chill.

Pour over ice in glasses, top up with a little sparkling water for a fizzy version or a garnish with slices of watermelon, raspberries or lemon wedges if desired and serve.

BLACKBERRY MOGITO ICE WATER

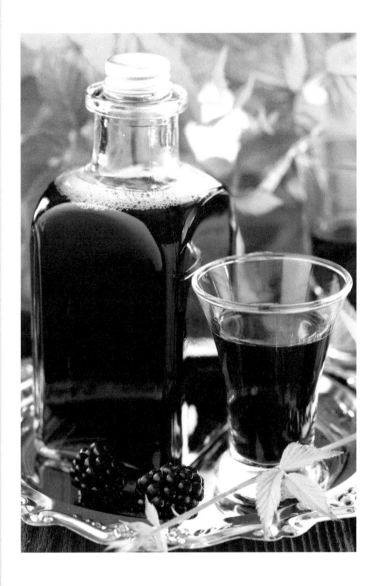

Ingredients:

1 quart of naturally alkalized spring water
5 organic blackberries
12 mint leaves
1 to 2 tablespoons manuka honey
1/2 fresh squeezed lime
1-1/2 ounces red herbal wine
Or 100% grape juice with natural
sweeteners (no high fructose corn syrup)

Directions:

Add ingredients into water pitcher, add water, allow mix to sit for 2 to 4 hours. Add ice. Garnish with a lime wheel, blackberry and a couple mint leaves. Serve and enjoy.

TROPICAL BRIGHT SANGRIA

Ingredients

2 blood oranges, halved and thinly sliced
2 kiwis, peeled and cut into wedges
1 cup seedless red grapes, halved or whole
1 mango, cut into bite-size pieces
2 bottles sauvignon blanc wine, chilled
2 ounces orange liqueur, such as Cointreau
8 ounces fresh strawberries, hulled and halved

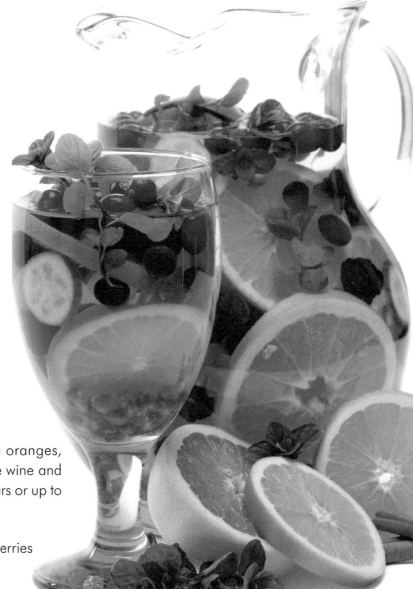

Directions

In a 1/2-gal. pitcher, combine the oranges, kiwis, grapes and mango. Stir in the wine and liqueur. Refrigerate for at least 2 hours or up to 6 hours.

Just before serving, stir in the strawberries

HOT LEMON DIURETIC KIDNEY CLEANSE

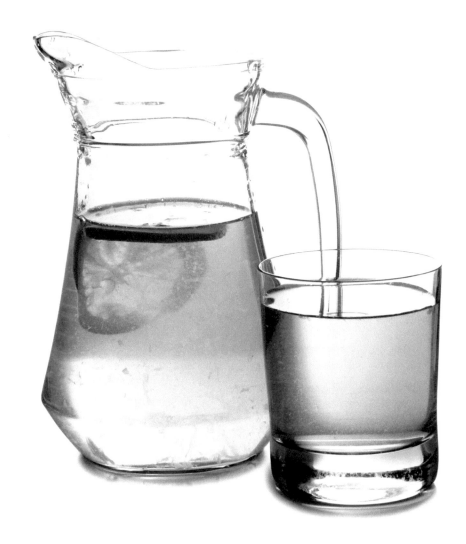

Makes two cups of hot Water.
2 organic lemons
Hot water

Put water in to teapot. Boil water, squeeze 2 lemons in to teapot. After you've squeezed all juice in, throw all four pieces into to teapot, keep the skins on. Lower temperature on the stove. Let this sit for about 2 minutes. Pour in to teacup. Drink up!

TANGERINE CUCUMBER AND STRAWBERRY INFUSED WATER

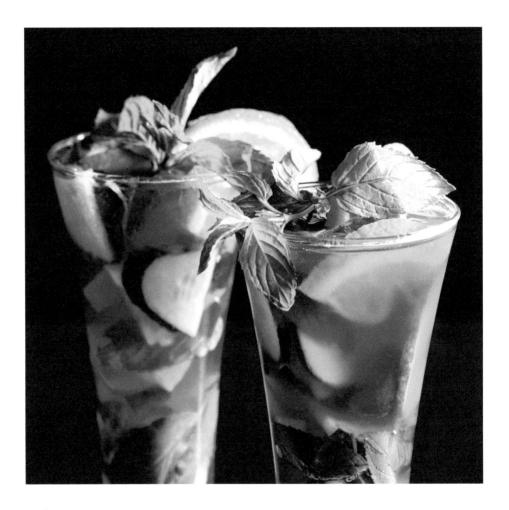

Ingredients; Makes 2 Liters

2 tangerines or 1 large orange, thinly sliced
5 inch cucumber, sliced into rings
10 strawberries, sliced into rings
2 cups of ice
Pitcher of pure alkalized spring Water

Mixing ingredients; add the tangerines, cucumber and strawberries. Top with ice and water. Let the pitcher sit in the fridge for 1 hour before serving.

When the water is down to 1/4 full in the pitcher, refill with water and place back in the fridge. You can do this several times with this Tangerine, Cucumber and Strawberry Infused Water. Store in the fridge up to 24 hours.

ORANGE STRAWBERRY MINT INFUSED WATER

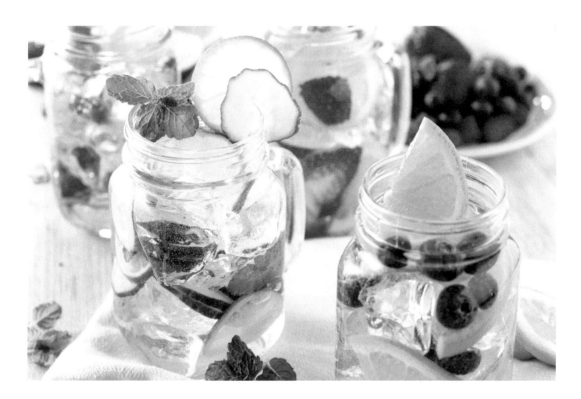

Ingredients

2 Orange
15 Strawberries, sliced
4 sprigs of fresh mint, about 16-20 leaves

Instructions:

Place 2 sliced oranges and 15 sliced strawberries into a large pitcher, which is the orange strawberry mix.

While holding the mint over the pitcher, begin to squeeze and stwist the mint, do not twist the mint too hard, gently enough to release the oils, then add the mint leaves to the fruit.

Let the mix within the pitcher sit at room temperature for 2 to 4 hours, then add ice and refrigerate for 1 hour before serving.

When the fruit water is down to ¼ , refill with natural spring water and place back in the refrigerator. You can do this several times.

When the water is all gone, you can make a smoothie with the strawberries, pealed oranges, and other ingredients, such as raspberries, lemons, and cucumbers.

GINGER ORANGE FRUIT INFUSED WATER

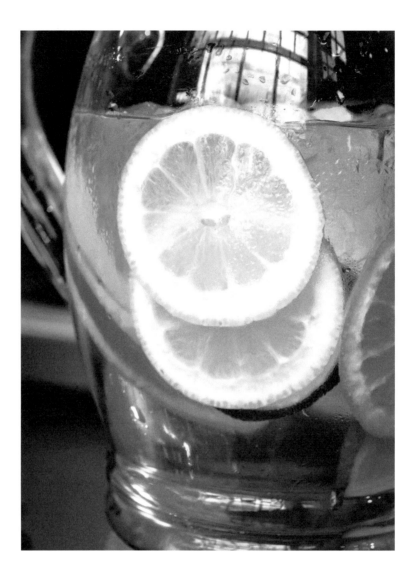

Ingredients:

The following recipe makes 1 liter, so if you have a 2 liter container double the ingredients, and so on.

½ orange
1 inch chunk of ginger
½ cup ice
1 table spoon of manuka honey
liter of pure alkalized spring water

Mix ingredients with in pitcher with one liter of water, add honey and stir until dissolved, allow to sit at room temperature for 2 to 4 hours, add ½ a cup of ice, serve and enjoy.

GINGER CINNAMON PEAR FRUIT WATER

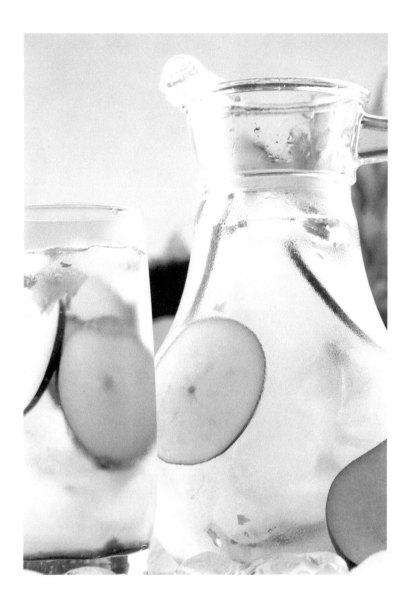

Ingredients:

1 ginger
1 cinnamon stick (or roll)
4 pears, sliced

Directions: Mix ingredients with in pitcher with one gallon of water, add honey and stir until dissolved, allow to sit at room temperature for 2 to 4 hours, place in the refrigerator, serve and enjoy.

CINNAMON AND HONEY COOL TEA

Ingredients:

Pitcher of natural alkaline spring water(gallon)
4 teaspoons Manuka honey
2 Cinnamon sticks (or rolls)

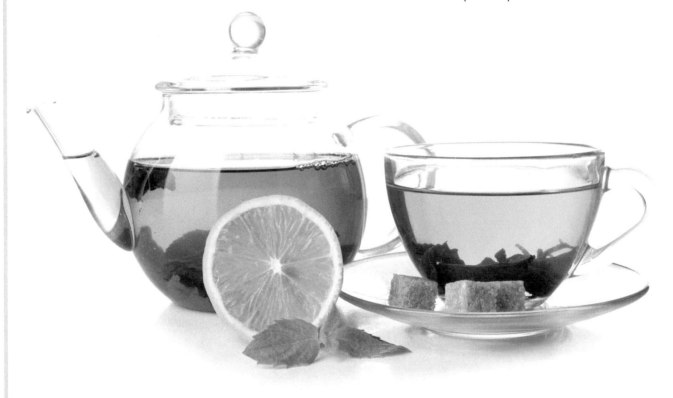

Directions: Mix ingredients with in pitcher with one gallon of water, add honey and stir until dissolved, allow to sit at room temperature for 2 to 4 hours, add ice, stir and serve… enjoy this cool and refreshing drink.

Cinnamon is good for reversing diabetes…

WATERMELON IS GREAT IN ASSISTING WITH HYDRATING THE BODY

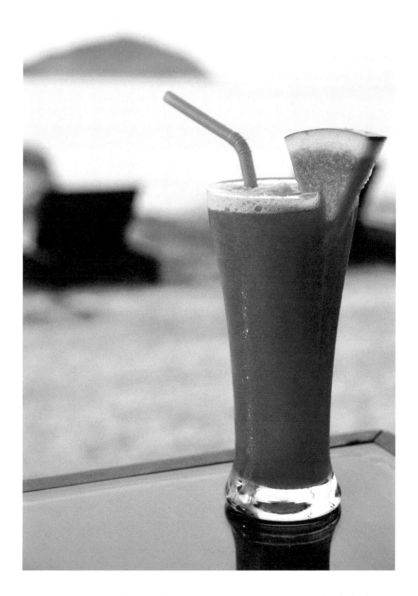

Watermelons are an excellent source of several vitamins too: vitamin A, which helps maintain eye health and is an antioxidant; vitamin C, which helps strengthens immunity, heal wounds, prevent cell damage, promote healthy teeth and gums; and vitamin B6, which helps brain function and helps convert protein to energy.

THE SIGNS OF DEHYDRATION

When the body suffers from acute or sever dehydration, the blood flow and blood pressure drop due to a lack of water and oxygen in the blood. Dehydration results when the body loses more water than it has taken in. Naturally this will cause the muscles and nerve function to literally burn out due in part to profuse sweating after exertion. How ever you can become dehydrated without any physical exercise.

If you have the stomach flu, and are suffering from water loss (due to a combination of vomiting and/or diarrhea) you will often feel fatigued. This is why doctors will recommend plenty of rest along with plenty of fluids, like water, juice, and herbal teas to replenish lost water levels.

Very dark, yellow urine is a first sign of dehydration. This typically occurs when blood pressure levels fall and the kidneys attempt to store water instead of expel it from the body. Dark urine describes urine that is a deeper than normal color. Although, for some dark urine is brown or deep yellow. For others it can appear maroon versus it's normal golden straw to yellow coloring.

Keep in mind that urine can change in color due a variety of reasons, dehydration being one of the most common. However, urine can be discolored due to medications, certain foods (i.e., beets), or such as a side effect of health conditions (i.e., liver disease). If you're urine is still discolored after you have hydrated and for no other apparent reason, talk to your doctor.

Dehydration often causes plummeting electrolyte levels, which will lead to increased heart rate, heart palpitations (or spasms) in the actual heart muscle. As blood pressure plummets, breathing and heart rate will quicken to indicate potential dehydration.

If you suspect you or someone you know is dehydrated, you can take their pulse and blood pressure reading lying down and again standing up. Take it for one minute each time as blood pressure will naturally drop a few seconds if you go from laying down to standing. Inadequate fluid in the blood will cause dehydration, quickening the heart rate and causing dizziness as inadequate blood is flowing to the brain. A quick heart rate check can be a good determinant of dehydration severity.

Fluid levels within the body keep our temperatures regulated so we don't become dehydrated and overheat— or even worse suffer dangerous heatstroke! However, thirst can send mixed signals when the body needs water. If your body needs a fluid level top up, it may often register as hunger. drink enough water, causing you to believe you need to eat when you really need to top up your liquid intake.

Obviously, if you are overheated due to physical exertion, you may become dehydrated due to fluid loss due to excessive perspiration. You can also suffer fluid loss from being in a hot environment.

That's why it's important to bring water(natural water) along with you if you plan to work out in a hot environment (i.e., hot yoga) or if you are outdoors in the heat and sun for even brief periods of time.

Hydration, or more so electrolyte balance, is vital for muscle contraction so when sodium and potassium stores are low it can cause painful muscle spasms. A muscle cramp (or spasm) will occur when a forcibly contracted (or involuntarily) muscle can't relax. We're used to contracting and controlling our muscles, but muscle, or even a few fibers of muscle, can contract or spasm involuntarily if fluid levels are low. Fluid levels are critical to the body functions.

Often dehydration will lead turn from muscle spasms to muscle cramps. This occurs when muscles contract and harden for a period of time that can last between a few seconds to hours. Muscle cramping with dehydration often occurs in the side (often called an abdominal stitch) or in a calf muscle. Both can be very painful, but hydrating can ease the pain and prevent continued cramping. Other than water fruits with potassium is great for muscle cramps.

 Water is necessary for efficient digestion, which means water absorption is required for healthy bowel movements. Fluids in your body help things along, including helping the food you eat move smoothly along your intestines and out of the body via bowel movements. Water also keep the intestinal walls smooth and malleable. That's why when we're dehydrated, the colon can become less flexible, contract slower, absorb less water, and result in stool (or body waste) that's hard, dry, and painful to pass.

Dehydration is a very common culprit of chronic constipation. Inadequate water levels in the body causes the large intestine to suck up water from your food waste, robbing stool of moisture. Keep your digestive system functioning normally and your bowel movements easy to pass by drinking plenty of fluids daily, and also by eating fiber, and getting regular exercise.

Listen to your body! One definite way to tell if you're dehydrated is when you're thirsty, your mouth and throat are dry, your tongue may feel sticky or dry, and even parched and swell in cases of extreme dehydration.

However, if you leave drinking until you feel thirsty, you may become dehydrated before you're actually thirsty. Thirst often sends confusing signals to the body and brain. For instance, you may feel hunger when dehydrated, which explains why a University of Washington study indicated that a single glass of water can easily shut down nighttime hunger pangs in almost all cases. However, "dry mouth," which is a dry, parched, thick feeling in the mouth can signal late stage of Dehydration.

Thank you for reading 'Pure Alkalized Fruit Water' and I sincerely hope that this book can be of an assistants to you ~ on your journey to balance your body's pH, by getting alkalized, to also assist in detoxing your body, increasing your energy, and purifying your sustaining substance of life, your own water ~ fasting and eating less starchy foods is a great path to take in cleansing the human body. Peace, and may you tap into the fountain of youth.

Printed in the United States
By Bookmasters